Essential Oils for Weight Loss

The Ultimate Beginners Guide to Lose Weight and Feel Great with Essential Oils

Copyright 2015 by Scott Jenkins - All rights reserved.

This document is geared towards providing exact and reliable information in regards to the topic and issue covered. The publication is sold with the idea that the publisher is not required to render accounting, officially permitted, or otherwise, qualified services. If advice is necessary, legal or professional, a practiced individual in the profession should be ordered.

- From a Declaration of Principles which was accepted and approved equally by a Committee of the American Bar Association and a Committee of Publishers and Associations.

In no way is it legal to reproduce, duplicate, or transmit any part of this document in either electronic means or in printed format. Recording of this publication is strictly prohibited and any storage of this document is not allowed unless with written permission from the publisher. All rights reserved.

The information provided herein is stated to be truthful and consistent, in that any liability, in terms of inattention or otherwise, by any usage or abuse of any policies, processes, or directions contained within is the solitary and utter responsibility of the recipient reader. Under no circumstances will any legal responsibility or blame be held against the publisher for any reparation, damages, or monetary loss due to the information herein, either directly or indirectly.

Respective authors own all copyrights not held by the publisher.

The information herein is offered for informational purposes solely, and is universal as so. The presentation of the information is without contract or any type of guarantee assurance.

The trademarks that are used are without any consent, and the publication of the trademark is without permission or backing by the trademark owner. All trademarks and brands within this book are for clarifying purposes only and are the owned by the owners themselves, not affiliated with this document.

Introduction

I want to thank you and congratulate you for purchasing the book, *"Essential Oils for Weight Loss: The Ultimate Beginners Guide to Lose Weight and Feel Great with Essential Oils."*

This book contains proven steps and strategies for losing weight through the use of essential oils. Also included in this book are weight loss recipes and helpful information about essential oils that specifically target weight issues.

Perhaps, one of the most sought after physical traits is the hourglass figure. It's the body shape that spells physical perfection. To achieve this figure, many turn to supplements that claim to melt away fat quicker than you can jog around the block. However, many users find that the short- and long-term side effects that accompany these "weight loss miracles" aren't worth the results. The exotic ingredients contained in weight loss supplements that consumers couldn't hope to pronounce are giving them a lot of eyebrow-raising doubt.

Keeping quality health in mind, more and more people turn to all-natural methods to lose weight fast. In recent years, aromatherapy has quickly become a favorite weight loss treatment among those who give alternative medicine a try. Backed by years of scientific research and tons of clinical trials, essential oils are becoming a fad in the world of health-conscious individuals. Due to their extensive health benefits, they are increasingly being explored by the scientific community. At this rate, synthetic drugs may soon become a thing of the past. As the pure essence of plants, essential oils are safe to use and virtually free of adverse side effects. To hold a vial of essential oil in the palm of your hand is to hold nature's pure botanical essence.

One ideal property of essential oils is their ability to induce weight loss by suppressing cravings, eliminating toxins, boosting metabolism, and reducing water retention. A healthy diet and regular exercise are catalysts that actually enhance the effects of essential oils. Whether you tip the scale or your pants don't fit as well around your waist as they used to, there's an essential oil within the pages of this book that's perfect for you. All you have to do is take a leap of faith and allow nature to treat you.

Thanks again for purchasing this book. I hope you enjoy it!

Chapter 1: Melt Away Fat with Citrus Essential Oils

Essential oils are extensively used in aromatherapy to treat various diseases and health conditions. Aromatherapy is an ancient Chinese method of healing that implements aromas to treat illnesses and promote overall health. There are over 90 essential oils used in aromatherapy. This book, however, only focuses on the oils that induce weight loss. While the number of essential oils for this particular purpose is still on the hefty side, this book aims to aid you in selecting the perfect oil by categorizing them according to aroma. To begin, we will first explore essential oils of the citrus category.

Grapefruit Essential Oil
Grapefruits are low-calorie fruits that are rich in vitamin C and powerful antioxidants, making them a great addition to diets designed with weight loss in mind. The fruit actually curbs your appetite by inducing a sensation of

satiety. Surprisingly, simply inhaling the aroma of grapefruit essence works just as well as a weight loss aid.

Grapefruit essential oil is derived from the rind of subtropical grapefruits. It contains roughly 90% limonene, the main active ingredient that gives the oil its weight loss properties. Limonene works by releasing fatty acids into your bloodstream, which your body metabolizes and uses for energy. Aside from increasing energy, grapefruit essential oil also suppresses appetite - particularly sugar cravings - dissolves fat, and prevents both bloating and water retention. Furthermore, it detoxifies your body when consumed; thus, eliminating harmful toxins that negatively influence weight. As an added benefit, the oil also reduces the appearance of cellulite.

Tons of research proved the effectiveness of grapefruit essential oil as a weight loss aid. One study investigated the aroma's weight loss effects on lab rats. When rats were introduced to the scent of grapefruit oil, they responded with a decrease in appetite and significant fat loss. Limonene, the researchers concluded, is the active chemical responsible for the loss of body fat in the lab rats.

How to Use

There are many ways to use grapefruit essential oil in aromatherapy as a weight loss aid. The best thing about the oil is that it's safe to take internally, applied topically, or inhaled. No unwanted side effects have been reported from ingesting or absorbing grapefruit essential oil.

1. **Diffusion:** You may consider infusing your home or office with its aroma with a diffuser while also decreasing your caloric intake by 250 calories - a small price to pay to enhance the weight loss effects of grapefruit essential oil.

2. **Supplement:** As previously mentioned, grapefruit essential oil is safe enough to ingest. In fact, consuming the oil is the quickest way to introduce limonene into your bloodstream. Once limonene

reaches your lymphatic system, it will cleanse the system of toxins that are stored in excess fat. The result? Loss of body fat and an increased metabolism. Simply switching out your morning cup o' Joe or ritualistic cup of orange juice with a glass of grapefruit water makes a world of difference.

Make a daily supplemental beverage by putting a drop or two of grapefruit essential oil in a glass of mineral water. Drink this simple, but invigorating, concoction every morning before breakfast. By doing so, you can give your body the fuel it needs to flush out toxins from your metabolic pathways and increase its fat-burning ability.

3. **Massage:** Grapefruit essential oil is highly absorbable by your skin. So if your taste buds aren't a fan of the grapefruit flavor, using the oil in a massage is the next best thing.

The high concentration of essential oils may not sit well with sensitive skin. This hurdle is easily surpassed by combining grapefruit oil with an ounce of a carrier oil. Studies show that olive oil is the best choice as it blends well with grapefruit oil and helps you consume less calories.

One or two drops of grapefruit essential oil for every ounce of carrier oil is all you need. Massage the mixture into the areas of your body where fat tends to accumulate for 30 minutes. It's important to refrain from washing the oil off for 3-4 hours so as to give your problem areas enough time to absorb all the goodness of the essential oil.

4. **Cellulite Bath:** Basking in the ambience of grapefruit essential oil offers relief from persistent subcutaneous fat known as cellulite. When your skin has areas with underlying fat deposits, it causes an

unsightly dimpled, lumpy appearance. Cellulite occurs primarily on the hips, thighs, and buttocks, which makes wearing a bikini difficult. Combat this problem today with the recipe below:

Ingredients:
- 6 drops of grapefruit essential oil
- 5 drops of orange essential oil
- 5 drops of ginger essential oil
- 5 drops of sandalwood essential oil
- 5 drops of lemon essential oil
- 1 cup of apple cider vinegar

Directions:
1. Add all the ingredients to a warm bath, making sure to disperse the essential oils well.

2. Soak for at least half an hour while massaging your problem areas.

Safety Precautions

Grapefruit essential oil is certainly edible, but there are a few safety issues to keep in mind. If you're taking medications to lower cholesterol levels or blood pressure, grapefruit may not be the oil for you as it interferes with these medications. Consult with your doctor first before incorporating grapefruit essential oil into your diet. Play it safe by using the oil in a diffuser instead of a daily supplement.

You can purchase Grapefruit Essential Oils here:

http://www.essentialoilenlightenment.com/GrapefruitOil

Lemon Essential Oil

Just like grapefruit, lemon essential oil has a high content of both vitamin C and limonene. In line with this, lemon produces a burst of energy and improve digestive health when inhaled. Because lemon essential oil contains limonene, it's a great detoxifying agent to flush out toxins from your fat cells. It's also an effective appetite suppressant.

For some, intestinal parasites that manage to go unnoticed may cause unwanted weight gain. Lemon essential oil gets rid of any secret parasites that may be lurking in your stomach.

How to Use
1. If there are areas on your body where fat accumulates, massaging lemon essential oil into these problem areas can eliminate the dimpling appearance caused by cellulite. Due to the unique molecular structure of the oil, your skin in these areas can easily absorb the weight-reducing nutrients that lemon essential oil has to offer.

When you free your body of harmful toxins, it will become leaner and healthier.

2. For a gentle detoxifying drink, dilute two drops of lemon essential oil in your daily drinking water. Drinking water enhanced with lemon oil every morning before a balanced breakfast will also speed up your metabolism, thereby increasing the rate through which you lose weight.

3. To curb your appetite and eliminate cravings, simply inhale the aroma of lemon essential oil whenever you're feeling particularly hungry.

Safety Precautions

Avoid applying lemon essential oil topically if you plan to be out in direct sunlight for long periods as lemon may increase the likelihood of sunburn. This is especially true for fair skin. In addition, while lemon essential oil is safe in both food and medicinal amounts, it's advisable to talk to your doctor about consuming more than two drops at a time.

You can purchase Lemon Essential Oils here:

http://www.essentialoilenlightenment.com/LemonOil

Bergamot Essential Oil

Bergamot essential oil is one of the all-time favorite oils among aromatherapy practitioners. Its sweet aroma contains hints of both fruit and floral, making it an ideal scent for most.

If stress-induced overeating is an issue, bergamot can help. It's common for those who suffer from weight issues to eat more during periods of emotional stress. As a science-backed mood enhancer, bergamot essential oil combats stress-related weight gain. Due to its sedative and antidepressant properties, the oil controls overeating triggered by stress. In fact, bergamot essential oil is one of the most commonly recommended alternative treatments for depression, anxiety, and chronic stress.

Bergamot essential oil is also perfect for those who have bad cholesterol due to its digestive properties. With a high content of the potent antioxidants known as polyphenols, bergamot oil is an effective substance for fighting oxidative damage. By inhibiting the production of fat in the bloodstream, bergamot increases metabolism while inhibiting your body's cholesterol absorption. Furthermore, bergamot can block enzymes that influence blood sugar levels in negative ways. As a result, your body more readily decomposes sugar and saturated fats.

How to Use

1. For an instant remedy for stress, put two drops of bergamot essential oil in a handkerchief. Whenever you're feeling stressed and thus, tempted to eat more, simply place the bergamot-scented handkerchief to your nose and inhale the vapors. Tuck it away in your pocket until the next use.

2. Enhance the calming effects of bergamot essential oil by combining it with coconut milk. Coconut is a great source of healthy fatty acids that promote fat loss. Prepare a soothing beverage by adding one or two drops of bergamot oil to a cup of warm coconut milk. Drink this

concoction any time stress tempts you to turn to food.

3. Bergamot essential oil is safe enough to take every day. For a subtle daily supplement, add a drop of the essential oil to a teaspoon of honey and consume each morning.

4. You can also dilute two drops of bergamot essential oil in an ounce of pure coconut oil, and massage the mixture into the back of your neck or your feet. Doing so practically melts the stress away due to the aroma it exudes.

5. For stress management, start your mornings with a quick 20-minute bath that includes ten drops of bergamot essential oil.

Safety Precautions
Bergamot essential oil is intended for adult use only. Since it's a highly concentrated substance, it is not recommended for children. Large amounts of bergamot can cause serious

side effects in children. Bergamot essential oil should not be used during pregnancy.

You can purchase Bergamot Essential Oil here:

http://www.essentialoilenlightenment.com/BergamotOil

Chapter 2: Camphoraceous Essential Oils are Slimming

Essential oils are described as being camphoraceous if they share similar properties as a chemical compound called camphor. The essential oils of the camphoraceous category have a unique, agreeable odor and a warm, semi-bitter taste.

<u>Peppermint Essential Oil</u>
Peppermint has a vast repertoire of health-promoting effects including relief from cramps, gas, indigestion, diarrhea, heartburn, and nausea. Aside from promoting digestive health, peppermint essential oil is also an extremely effective anti-inflammatory agent that treats headaches, nerve pain, and toothaches.

As an essential oil, peppermint aids in weight loss endeavors particularly by reducing appetite and suppressing cravings for sweets and junk food. What's more, the oil also eliminates stress-eating. Peppermint essential oil works by operating on the area of the brain responsible for triggering the feeling of being full during meals. By affecting your brain's satiety center, peppermint essential oil enables you to eat less and still feel satisfied.

Furthermore, peppermint has been found to be the most effective aroma for stimulating the production of a specialized neurotransmitter known as serotonin, which is linked to the "sweet tooth" phenomenon.

The simple act of deep inhalation of peppermint essential oil is a science-backed method for weight loss. This was demonstrated by a clinical trial in which test subjects were exposed to the aroma of peppermint essential oil while some were not. The study confirmed the appetite-suppressing effects of inhaling the aroma of peppermint oil. Participants who inhaled the aroma felt less hunger pangs and had significantly fewer cravings than those who didn't.

It's impossible to go wrong with peppermint essential oil. Even when you've reached your weight loss goals, continuous use of the oil will help with weight maintenance. Since it's chock full of omega-3 fatty acids, vitamins, magnesium, and iron, peppermint essential oil doesn't just end with weight loss: it nourishes your body and promotes an ongoing sense of well-being, thereby keeping you in peak health.

How to Use
1. To curb your appetite between meals, simply open a vial of peppermint essential oil and deeply inhale the aroma it exudes. The unique camphoraceous, sweet-smelling scent of the oil is powerful enough to stop cravings.

2. To avoid overeating, drink a glass of cool water infused with two drops of peppermint essential oil during or before a meal. Be sure to use high quality, food grade peppermint oil that is safe for internal use.

3. Make a clever on-the-go diffuser by adding two drops of peppermint essential oil onto a cotton ball. Seal

the fluffy ball in a small zip-lock bag and take it with you wherever you go. Whenever you're feeling particularly hungry, simply take the cotton ball out and slowly inhale its aroma.

4. For an energizing morning shower, add 5 drops of peppermint essential directly on the floor of your shower. When hot water hits your shower floor, your whole bathroom will be diffused with the invigorating scent of peppermint. The hot water will also open up your pores, allowing the peppermint-infused steam to penetrate into your skin. As a byproduct, you'll notice a marked reduction in cravings for high-calorie breakfast foods like sausages, bacon, muffins, donuts, and pancakes.

Other camphoraceous essential oils you can use for their weight loss benefits include marjoram, eucalyptus, and rosemary. The aroma these essential oils exude is deeply penetrating, thus stimulating healing and weight loss more readily.

You can purchase Peppermint Essential Oil here:

http://www.essentialoilenlightenment.com/YLPeppermintOil

Chapter 3: Spicy and Woody Essential Oils for Weight Loss

Essential oils of the spicy and woody class give you a burst of energy which, in turn, impacts your weight. Most oils with woody aromas are known to relax and uplift. In this chapter, we will take a look at essential oils that exude spicy/woody aromas for weight loss.

Cinnamon Essential Oil

Known as the oldest spice still being used in modern times, cinnamon essential oil has been used for its therapeutic effects for hundreds of years. This is yet another essential oil that acts as both a metabolism booster and appetite suppressant. Cinnamon essential oil inhibits your body from storing sugars as fat. Instead, the oil stimulates your body to convert sugars into energy. As a result, your body has less fats to store.

Another great benefit of cinnamon essential oil is the ability of its sweet-and-spicy aroma to induce a premature feeling of fullness during meals. Because of this effect, cinnamon essential oil is great for any weight loss plan as well as weight maintenance regimens. Even better, cinnamon acts as an enhancer that boosts the effects of other essential oils used for weight loss. It even increases libido as an added benefit.

How to Use
1. While there are countless cinnamon-based weight loss recipes out there, the one below is the most commonly used:

Ingredients:

- 2 drops of cinnamon essential oil
- 1 teaspoon of good quality honey
- 1 cup of water

Directions:
1. Start by bringing one cup of water to a boil in a small saucepan or microwave.

2. In a cup, combine the cinnamon essential oil and honey, and mix well.
3. Add the boiling water to the cinnamon-honey mixture and let it sit for 30 minutes or until cooled.
4. Stir well and drink half of the concoction on an empty stomach right before breakfast.
5. Refrigerate the rest and drink it before bedtime.

Using this recipe regularly can help you shed at least two pounds by the end of the week. Once you've reached your weight loss goals, you can continue drinking this cinnamon-honey beverage for the perfect weight maintenance plan.

2. For a quick appetite suppressant, drink two drops of bergamot essential oil diluted in a glass of water. This cinnamon-flavored

drink works best when consumed half an hour before each meal.

3. To eliminate hunger pangs throughout the day, simply inhale the aroma of cinnamon essential oil through your diffuser.

You can purchase Cinnamon Essential Oils here:

http://www.essentialoilenlightenment.com/CinnamonOil

Sandalwood Essential Oil

Due in part to sharing the same aroma class as cinnamon, sandalwood essential oil also lifts your spirits and improves mood. In this way, sandalwood helps in your weight loss efforts by enabling you to overcome stress-related eating. By eliminating negative feelings that accompany stress, sandalwood essential oil helps get rid of the temptation to eat more to deal with emotional stress. Furthermore, the woodsy aroma of sandalwood can reduce tension and confusion. It also provides a harmonizing effect. Even better, sandalwood essential is one of the safest weight loss aids as it is nontoxic, non-sensitizing, and non-irritant.

How to Use

1. **Vaporizer:** Vaporization is one of the best ways to enjoy sandalwood essential oil. There are countless vaporizers in the market, with the most ideal ones being glass and terracotta. By vaporizing an essential oil, you get both the

benefit of an aromatic room and therapeutic effects.

If you opt to vaporize sandalwood essential oil for weight loss use, do it properly. The vaporizer you buy should have a large top reservoir. Eight drops of sandalwood oil are sufficient enough to bring a spicy, woody, stress-relieving fragrance to a large living room.

2. **Daily supplement:** As with most essential oils, you can take a drop of sandalwood oil every morning with a teaspoon of honey.

3. **Massage:** Dilute one drop of sandalwood essential oil in an ounce of coconut oil and rub the mixture into your stomach. A simple hand or feet massage works great, too.

Sandalwood essential oil blends well with lavender and bergamot oil. Consider making a fragrant massage oil blend using one drop each of sandalwood, lavender, and bergamot essential oil with two ounces of coconut oil. Massage the mixture into your wrists to enjoy the stress-relieving effects of all three oils.

You can purchase Sandalwood Essential Oil here:

http://www.essentialoilenlightenment.com/SandalwoodOil

Ginger Essential Oil

Nutritionists generally agree that ginger is one of the best things to put in your body if you want to lose weight. Ginger oil actually increases the rate at which your body burns fat, making it an ideal complement to routine exercise. When used internally, ginger essential oil increases metabolism and improves the overall function of your digestive system. It even works as an effective weight loss aid when applied topically as it reduces both the appearance and occurrence of subcutaneous fat. Ginger essential oil is a perfect suppressant for cravings as well.

In general, the more ginger you incorporate into your diet, the easier it will be to lose weight. This is due to the ginger's ability to support digestion and facilitate the absorption of essential nutrients from the food you eat.

The best way to use ginger essential oil as a weight loss aid is to consume it. If you can tolerate the strong aroma and taste of the oil, put a drop under your tongue. If not, feel free to dilute a drop or two in a glass of juice or water. While topical application isn't as effective, the fat-reducing effect of ginger essential oil is certainly beneficial when used in massage therapy. Like with all essential oils, it's important to dilute ginger oil in a carrier oil.

You can purchase Ginger Essential Oils here:

http://www.essentialoilenlightenment.com/GingerOil

Chapter 4: DIY Weight Loss Recipes

There are countless essential oil recipes for weight loss. This chapter lists some of the most widely used recipes that, when accompanied with a healthy lifestyle, will enable you to reach your weight loss goals.

Keep in mind that essential oils are dense and highly concentrated. If you plan on applying essential oils topically, avoid doing so in their undiluted form. Dilute the essential oil first with a carrier oil of your choice to make the oil mild enough for topical application.

Ultimate Essential Oil Blend

This blend takes four key essential oils and combines their powerful effects into one effective oil blend for shedding body fat. If your budget doesn't allow for a visit to an aromatherapist, this blend is a relatively inexpensive alternative—and incredibly easy to make, too.

Ingredients:

- 5 drops of peppermint essential oil
- 10 drops of bergamot essential oil
- 10 drops of sandalwood essential oil
- 15 drops of grapefruit essential oil
- A ceramic bowl
- A clean spoon
- A dark tinted glass vial
- Carrier oil as needed

Directions:

1. Start by combining all of the essential oils in a clean bowl, and mix well.
2. Carefully pour the blend into a vial. Shake well.
3. Use ten drops of the blend for every bath, making sure to soak for at least 30 minutes while massaging the areas of your body where fat tends to accumulate.
4. For a quick massage, simply dilute 1-2 drops of the essential oil blend in an ounce of almond, jojoba, coconut, or extra virgin olive oil. Massage the mixture into your

cellulite-prone areas, your forehead, the back of your neck, or your feet.
5. This special blend also works great in your diffuser. 6-8 drops should do the trick.

Cellulite and Anti-Fattening Trio Cream

Eliminating excess fat and reducing the appearance of cellulite will make a huge difference in your weight loss endeavors. Skip the synthetic substances and harsh chemicals; instead, make your own homemade cream with just a couple of ingredients.

All you have to do is choose one of the essential oils listed in this book and mix 10 drops in a small bottle of unscented lotion or moisturizing cream. You'll get all the benefits of skin nourishment plus the added therapeutic effects of the essential oil you choose. Whether you're trying to curb your hunger or get rid of toxins that cause a buildup of fat beneath your skin, this DIY cellulite and anti-fattening cream can help.

Weight Loss Shot

The last thing you need if you're trying to shed a few unwanted pounds is alcohol. However, this recipe allows you to take shots without harming your health. It includes absolutely zero alcohol—just the slimming and therapeutic benefits of three essential oils. This shot improves metabolism and digestion, significantly reduces stress, and wards off midday and midnight cravings. It offers approximately one week of use, so feel free to double or triple the ingredients for prolonged usage.

Ingredients:

- 5 drops of either grapefruit or lemon essential oil
- 5 drops of bergamot essential oil
- 5 drops of frankincense essential oil
- A tinted glass vial with dropper

Directions:

1. Add all three essential oils in a vial and shake to combine.
2. Fill a shot glass with water or fresh orange juice. Add 1-2 drops of the oil blend. Bottoms up!
3. Repeat three times a day before each meal, or anytime stress or cravings raise their ugly heads.

Slimming Beverage

This recipe combines five weight-reducing essential oils for the ultimate weight loss drink. It works great as an appetite suppressant, and is mild enough to drink throughout the day. In fact, it is recommended to drink this beverage as often as four times a day as essential oils are quickly absorbed and utilized by your body. Supplying your body with a consistent flow of essential oils is important for ultimate efficacy. This beverage also promotes sleep: proper rest is a key tool for any weight loss plan.

Ingredients:

- 20 drops of cinnamon essential oil (Make sure to use essential oil derived from cinnamon bark.)
- 40 drops of grapefruit essential oil
- 40 drops of lemon essential oil
- 40 drops of ginger essential oil
- 40 drops of peppermint essential oil
- A 15ml tinted glass vial with dropper

Directions:

1. Put all of the essential oils into a vial and shake to combine well. Your vial should be nearly full once you've added all of the ingredients.
2. Before each meal, dilute two drops of the oil blend in a glass cup of cool mineral water, and drink.

The Truth About Essential Oils Manufacturers

Many essential oils manufacturers skimp on the quality of their product in order to maximize their profit margin, as I'm sure you know this happens in virtually every industry... however when we're talking about products we're going to be inhaling, applying to our skin and in some cases ingesting its of paramount importance that we're using high quality oils and that we know exactly what we're getting!

After copious amounts of my own research and discussion with other essential oil enthusiasts I decided to try Young Living essential oils and have never looked backed since – Young Living are the absolute best and the leaders in the essential oil industry.

Check out this graphic below on 10 reasons why I use Young Living products.

10 Reasons To Choose Young Living™ Essential Oils

1. Young Living owns their own farms.
2. Anyone can visit farms and participate in the harvest and distillation process.
3. The Seed to Seal promise rocks.
4. YLEOs are first distillation oils ONLY.
5. Each batch of EO is rigourously tested in-house and via 3rd party testing.
6. Pest control is done with EOs.
7. Weed control is by hand.
8. Young Living has 20+ years of experience and research!
9. Young Living has the greatest selection of singles and blends available on the market!
10. The support, education and community that Oily Families provides make joining Young Living an incredible, empowering experience!

The Best Essential Oils Starter Kit, Ever

WHAT'S IN YOUR PREMIUM STARTER KIT?

SINGLES
- 1 – 5 ml Frankincense
- 1 – 5 ml Lemon
- 1 – 5 ml Lavender
- 1 – 5 ml Melaleuca Alternifolia (tea tree oil)
- 1 – 5 ml Peppermint

BLENDS
- 1 – 5 ml Joy™
- 1 – 5 ml Purification®
- 1 – 5 ml PanAway®
- 1 – 5 ml Thieves®
- 1 – 5 ml Stress Away™

ALSO INCLUDED!

In addition to these essential oils, your kit includes the following: a Home Diffuser, Welcome to Young Living booklet, Essential Oils at a Glance user's guide, Distributor Resource Guide, S.E.E.D. Sharing for Success booklet, Citrus Fresh 5-ml, AromaGlide Roller Fitment, two Lavender Sample Packets, two Peppermint Sample Packets, two Peace & Calming Sample Packets, two Lemon Sample Packets, two Thieves Sample Packets, Sample Packet Business Cards, two NingXia Red 2-oz. samples, Distributor Agreement, Product Guide and Product Price List.

The Young Living Premium Starter Kit contains all the everyday oils you'll get the most use out of and come to love! You even get a comprehensive user guide to ensure you're using all of the oils correctly. Eliminate the guesswork.

You'll get ten amazing oils including:

Lavender, Peppermint, Lemon, Frankiscence, PanAway, Copaiba, Thieves, Purification, R.C and DiGize + A bonus Stress Away.

<u>As well as…</u>

A beautiful diffuser to use at home (perfect for Peppermint!)

Aroma Glide roller fitment (to turn any oil into a roll on)

Two **sample packets** each of Lavender, Peppermint, Peace & Calming, Lemon, and Thieves

Two NingXia Red 2oz samples (an antioxidant drink concentrate that's a great supplement for supporting health and well being)

<u>Follow the link below and select 'Member' to orders yours now.</u>

<u>http://www.essentialoilenlightenment.com/buyoils</u>

Save 24% on all essential oils!

When you purchase your Young Living Premium Starter Kit you automatically become a "wholesale member" of Young Living.

This means you can continue to buy *other* Young Living products for a huge 24% discount off the retail price!

You're under zero obligation to buy any other products as a wholesale member, but if you do, you get 24% off!

http://www.essentialoilenlightenment.com/buyoils

and select '**Member**'.

Enter your details and ensure that the ID number **3064309** is present in the Sponsor ID and Enroller ID fields.

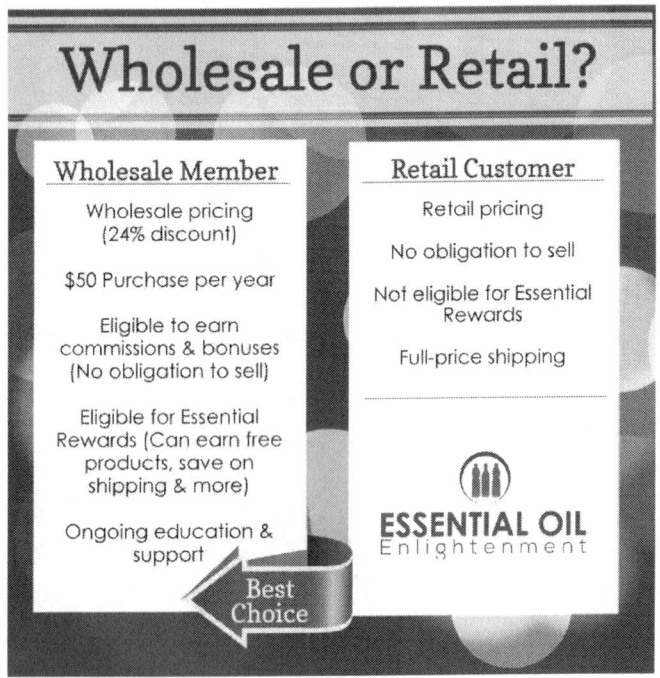

Conclusion

Thanks again for purchasing this book!

I hope this book was able to provide you with the knowledge of the best and the most effective essential oils to use in your weight loss endeavors.

One of the safest and most natural solutions to your weight-related woes is, quite literally, right under your nose. Making a conscious effort to use your powerful sense of smell gives you the capability to control your weight where your willpower fails. Whether you want to shed several pounds in a month or you're weight has plateaued, using the right essential oils can help you reach your weight loss goals. Essential oils are non-toxic and safe enough for prolonged use, allowing you to use them in your weight maintenance practices.

The next step is to apply everything you've learned in this book to your weight loss plan to speed up results. I hope you enjoy the essential oil recipes and that you succeed in your weight loss endeavors.

Thank you, and good luck!

Want To Read More?

Be sure to check out my blog for TONS more free information, recipes, benefits, how-to's and more with essential oils!

www.EssentialOilEnlightenment.com

See you there!

Scott Jenkins

Made in the USA
Lexington, KY
28 November 2017